Natural Treatments

for

Heart Diseases

Through Medicinal Alkaline Herbs, Diets, & Aerobic Physiotherapy that Boost Natural Immunity; Detoxification & Prevent Infections, Inflammation & Cardiac Arrest

Esther Gbemy

Table of Contents

Introduction

The heart is a muscular organ that draws deoxygenated blood from every area of the body, transports it to the lungs to remove carbon dioxide from the blood and subsequently add oxygen to the blood through breathing of fresh air in the surrounding. After which the blood is transported from the lungs back to the Heart and distributes it to every part of the body.

The heart is located right beneath the sternum, or breastbone, which joins your ribs at the center. It weighs around 300 grams (half a pound) and is about the size of your fist.

The heart of an adult beats between 60 and 80 times a minute, but the heart of a newborn baby beats between 70 and 190 times every minute, which is quicker than the heart of an adult.

The pericardium encloses the heart, which has a shape that is slightly conical. With one third on the right and two thirds on the left of the midline, it is positioned posterior to the body of the sternum. The heart weighs 310 g (for men) and 255 g (for females).

The center of the chest is where the heart is located, and it leans slightly to the left. Blood is pumped to every region of the body with each heartbeat. Every day, your heart beats around 100,000 times which is about 3 billion beats in a lifetime.

Anything short of this causes problems in the heart, which is regarded as heart diseases. Heart disease is the leading single factor that results to death worldwide. Heart disease in all of its forms is a crucial, life-or-death issue. Rather of being one illness, it is a collection of illnesses and trauma to the cardiovascular system (the heart and blood vessels).

Around the world, cardiovascular disease (CVD) is a key factor in disability and early mortality. Atherosclerosis is the underlying disease, which takes years to develop and is often advanced by the time symptoms appear, typically in middle age. Heart attacks and strokes are both unexpected, acute cerebrovascular episodes that usually result in death before medical attention can be offered.

In both those with pre-existing cardiovascular illness and those who are at high cardiovascular risk owing to one or more risk factors, risk factor reduction can lower clinical events and premature mortality. Most frequently, they are conditions affecting the heart and the blood arteries in the heart and brain.

A leading cardiologist claims that by the time a person is 35 years old, the majority of people who will develop a form of cardiovascular disease (CVD) already have the disease's early stages. Cardiovascular diseases (CVD) typically affect people in their later years (with incidence rising sharply after the 30-44 age range).

Heart disease may be prevented and reversed in large part by diet and lifestyle changes, and several herbs and supplements can help both reduce your chance of developing heart disease and cure existing issues.

The primary cause of most heart diseases, atherosclerosis, may be combated with the use of a number of herbs and vitamins. Plaque accumulates in your arteries as a result of atherosclerosis, preventing oxygen-rich blood from reaching your heart and other organs. It could potentially result in death or a heart attack.

The factors that cause heart diseases includes: High blood pressure, Smoking or exposure to secondhand smoke, Diabetes, High cholesterol…and more.

There are different traditional methods used in the treatment of heart problems, as there are different types of heart problems with different causes.

In the course of writing this book, I will show you different methods such as the use of therapeutic alkaline herbs, the employment of physiotherapy, especially for stroke patients and the consumption of healing diets that contains reduced amount of fat, cholesterol and acid contents.

I am very sure you will enjoy every bit of this book.

Chapter One

The Human Heart

The heart is a muscular organ that draws deoxygenated blood from every area of the body, transports it to the lungs for oxygenation, and then expels oxygen and carbon dioxide. The blood is then transported from the lungs and distributed to every part of the body.

The heart is a muscle located right beneath the sternum, or breastbone, which links your ribs. It weighs around 300 grams (half a pound) and is about the size of your fist.

The heart of an adult beats between 60 and 80 times a minute, but the heart of a newborn baby beats between 70 and 190 times every minute, which is quicker than the heart of an adult.

The blood travels to your lungs, where it absorbs oxygen, after leaving the right side of the heart. Once it has returned to your heart, the oxygen-rich blood is circulated through a system of arteries to the body's organs.

Veins carry the blood back to your heart, where it is then pushed to your lungs once more. Circulation is the term for this action.

The coronary arteries, a network of blood vessels on the surface of the heart, provide the heart with its own supply of blood.

The pericardium encloses the heart, which has a shape that is slightly conical. With one third on the right and two thirds on the left of the midline, it is positioned posterior to the body of the sternum. The heart weighs 310 g (for men) and 255 g (for females).

The left lung and pleura are located anteriorly, as well as the sternum's body and surrounding costal cartilages (apex).

The Oesophagus, descending thoracic aorta, azygos, hemiazygos veins, and thoracic duct are located posteriorly.

The Heart Walls' Layers

The pericardium encloses three layers of the heart wall:

- The visceral layer of the serous pericardium forms the epicardium, the outer layer of the heart's wall.

- Myocardium - the conducting system and excitable tissue are found in this muscular middle layer of the heart's wall.

- Endocardium - a center, circumferential layer an intracardiac layer.

Specifically, the subepicardial and subendocardial layers make up the majority of the remaining heart tissue.

The Heart's Structure in Brief

The right and left sides of the heart are separated by septa, and a constriction splits each half of the organ into two chambers; the top cavity is known as the atrium and the bottom cavity as the ventricle.

Consequently, the heart has four chambers:

- The right atrium.

- The left atrium.

- The right ventricle.

- The Left ventricle.

The sequence in which the four chambers and four valves are encountered by the blood as it passes through the heart is the one to remember:

The right atrium receives the body's venous blood in return. Blood is pumped from the right atrium into the right ventricle via the tricuspid valve.

Blood is pumped from the right ventricle into the pulmonary artery and then via the pulmonary semilunar valve to the lungs, where it is oxygenated.

The four pulmonary veins carry blood from the lungs back into the left atrium. Blood is pumped from the left atrium into the left ventricle via the bicuspid (mitral) valve.

The Heart Valves

Four heart valves are present. These include:

- Pulmonary valve: The right ventricle and the pulmonary artery are separated by the pulmonary valve. It enables blood to flow from the right ventricle to the pulmonary artery and then towards the lungs in a single route.

- The aorta: This is situated between the left ventricle and the aorta. It opens to let blood to flow from the left ventricle to the aorta in a single path.

- The mitral: This is situated between the left atrium and the left ventricle. It permits blood to go normally from the atrium to the ventricle in a single path.

- The tricuspid valve: this keeps the blood flowing properly. The valves only open in one direction when necessary. Valves must fully open and seal securely to prevent leaks. The right atrium and right ventricle are separated by the tricuspid valve. It enables blood to go from the right atrium to the right ventricle in a single route.

How Does the Heart Works?

Knowing how the heart functions may be useful in understanding the causes of cardiac disease.

- There are two upper chambers (atria) and two lower chambers in the heart (ventricles).

- Blood veins on the right side of the heart transport blood to the lungs (pulmonary arteries).

- Blood absorbs oxygen in the lungs before returning to the left side of the heart via the pulmonary veins.
- The blood is then pumped from the left side of the heart to the rest of the body through the aorta.

How Does the Heart beats?

A beating heart continuously cycles via contraction and relaxation.

The ventricles, the lower heart chambers, contract tightly during systole. Blood is compelled to the lungs and the rest of the body by this movement.

Blood from the upper heart chambers fills the ventricles during diastole (atria).

The Heart's Electrical System

The electrical circuitry in the heart keeps it beating. The constant interchange of oxygen-rich blood with oxygen-poor blood is managed by the heartbeat. You are kept alive by this transaction.

The lower cardiac chambers receive the impulses via specific channels (ventricles). It instructs the heart to beat.

Overview of Cardiovascular Disease

Cardiovascular disease (CVD) is a serious and life-or-death issue since it is the leading cause of mortality worldwide. The cardiovascular system is affected by a number of illnesses and traumas together known as CVD (the heart and blood vessels).

Most frequently, they are conditions affecting the heart and the blood arteries in the heart and brain. Although a top cardiologist claims that by the time a person is 35 years old, the majority of persons who will develop a type of CVD already have the disease's early stages, it is true that they typically afflict people in their later years (with incidence rising dramatically after the 30-44 age range).

Atherosclerosis, a buildup of fatty deposits inside the arteries, and a higher risk of blood clots are typically connected with it.

It may also be linked to artery damage in several organs, including the kidneys, eyes, heart, brain, and heart.

One of the biggest causes of mortality and disability in the United Kingdom is CVD, yet it is frequently significantly avoidable by adopting a healthy lifestyle.

Blood flow to the heart, brain, or other regions of the body may be limited by blood arteries that have constricted or been clogged as a result of cardiovascular disease.

Symptoms of Cardiovascular Disease

The symptoms of cardiovascular disease are:

- Coronary artery disease, which affects the main blood channels that supply the heart with blood, oxygen, and nutrients

- Cerebrovascular disease, a condition that affects the blood arteries that supply the brain.

- Peripheral artery disease: A illness that affects the blood arteries supplying the arms and legs.

- Rheumatic heart disease: Rheumatic fever, which is brought on by an infection with streptococcal bacteria, damages the heart muscle and heart valves.

- Congenital heart disease or congenital abnormalities of the heart.
- Pulmonary embolisms: Blood clots that originate in the leg veins and can get dislodged and go to the heart and lungs.

Heart attacks and strokes are serious medical illnesses mostly brought on by a blockage that stops blood from getting to the heart or brain.

The accumulation of fatty deposits on the inner walls of the blood arteries that supply the heart or brain is the most frequent cause of this obstruction. Strokes can also result from blood clots or bleeding from a brain blood vessel.

In many cases, there are no symptoms or warning indicators that someone has a cardiovascular illness.

- The first indication or symptom of the condition might be a heart attack or stroke.
- Chest pain or discomfort in the middle.

- Repulsion.

- Feeling dizzy or faint.

- Back or jaw discomfort, nausea, vomiting, and shortness of breath are more common in women.

- Arm, left shoulder, elbow, jaw, or back pain or discomfort.

- The patient may have trouble breathing or feel out of breath.

- Perspiring.

Chapter Two

Types of Heart Diseases

As previously established, cardiovascular disorders collectively make up the term "CVD."

These include aortic aneurysm and dissection, deep vein thrombosis, rheumatic heart disease, congenital heart disease, angina, stroke, coronary heart disease, and other, less prevalent cardiovascular conditions.

Stroke/Trascient Ischemic Attack (TIA)

When a portion of the brain's blood supply is cut off, a stroke occurs, which may result in death or severe brain damage.

Similar to a stroke, a transient ischemic attack (also known as a TIA or "mini-stroke") causes a brief disruption in the blood supply to the brain.

The area of the brain supplied by a blocked or burst artery is no longer able to receive the oxygen delivered by the blood; as a result, brain cells suffer damage or pass away (become necrotic), reducing that area of the brain's functionality. If a stroke is not immediately detected and treated, it may result in death or lasting brain damage.

Ischemic and hemorrhagic strokes fall into two main groups. Ischemia can result from systemic hypoperfusion, thrombosis (clotting), or embolism (clot or blockage from elsewhere in the body) (reduction of the blood flow to all parts of the body).

Subarachnoid or intracerebral hemorrhage are two causes of hemorrhage. Ischemic strokes account for 80% of cases.

The Primary Signs and Symptoms

The main symptoms of stroke are:

Face: The person's lips or eye may have dropped, their face may have drooped on one side, or they may not be able to smile.

Arms: Due to arm weakness or numbness in one arm, the person might not be able to elevate both arms and maintain them there.

Speech: They can be unable to speak at all, have slurred or garbled speech, or have trouble understanding what you are communicating to them.

Other symptoms include:

- An excruciating headache with no apparent explanation.
- Loss of consciousness or fainting.
- Numbness, often on one side of the body, in the face, arm, or leg.
- Facial, arm, or leg weakness that occurs suddenly, most frequently on one side of the body.
- Difficulty using one or both eyes to see.
- Trouble walking, lightheadedness, loss of balance, or lack of coordination.

What causes stroke?

Like all organs, the brain depends on blood's supply of nutrients and oxygen to function effectively. Brain cells start to die if the blood supply is reduced or interrupted.

This may result in a brain damage, incapacity, or even death.

Strokes have two basic causes:

Ischemic: 85% of cases are ischemic, in which the blood flow is interrupted by a blood clot.

Hemorrhagic: this is when a brain blood artery that is weak bursts.

What Causes Transient Ischemic Attack (TIA)?
One of the blood arteries that transport oxygen-rich blood to your brain becomes blocked during a TIA.

Although air bubbles or particles of fatty material can potentially cause this obstruction, the most common cause is a blood clot that developed elsewhere in your body and traveled to the blood veins supplying the brain.

Your risk of getting a TIA may be increased by certain factors, such as:

- Diabetic.
- Smoking.
- High Blood Pressure (Hypertension).
- Frequent irregular heartbeat.
- Obesity.

- High levels of Cholesterol

- Consuming huge amounts of alcohol.

Condition that increases ones risk of having stroke are:

- High cholesterol.

- High blood pressure.

- Diabetes.

- Irregular heartbeats.

Deep Vein Thrombosis

A blood clot (thrombus) that forms in a deep vein, typically in the lower leg, is known as a Deep Vein Thrombosis (DVT). Leg discomfort and probable consequences are two effects of deep vein thrombosis.

In the United Kingdom, 1-3 out of every 1000 persons experience Deep Vein Thrombosis. Although it can happen anywhere, including the arm, a Deep Vein Thrombosis often originates in a deep vein in the leg.

The muscles are all around the deep veins, which go through the middle of the leg. Blood clots that develop in a distinct set of veins under the skin (known as superficial veins) are different from Deep Vein Thrombosis. These less dangerous blood clots are known as superficial thrombophlebitis.

Although Deep Vein Thrombosis seldom leads to further issues, Pulmonary Embolism (PE) and post-thrombotic syndrome are two possible side effects. Pulmonary Embolism is brought on when a fragment of the blood clot separates, travels through the circulation, and becomes stuck in the lungs, blocking blood flow.

This may occur hours, days, or even longer after the clot in the leg veins has formed. Breathlessness and chest discomfort are possible side effects.

A Deep Vein Thrombosis can damage a vein's valves, causing the blood to pool in the lower leg rather than flow upward, which is known as post-thrombotic syndrome. Leg ulcers, soreness, and edema may arise from this.

Coronary Heart Disease

The buildup of atheromatous plaques inside the walls of the arteries that supply the myocardium causes coronary heart disease (CHD), also known as coronary artery disease (CAD) and atherosclerotic heart disease (the muscle of the heart).

The majority of people with coronary heart disease do not exhibit any symptoms or indications of the condition for decades as the disease advances before the first signs and symptoms, which are frequently a "sudden" heart attack, that eventually appear.

After decades of development, some of these atheromatous plaques may rupture and begin restricting blood flow to the heart muscle along with activating the blood clotting mechanism. The illness is the most frequent reason for unexpected death.

Coronary heart disease can result to the following:

- Angina (chest pain).
- Heart attack.
- Heart failure.

Causes of Coronary Heart Disease

The condition known as coronary heart disease is what occurs when a buildup of fatty substances in the coronary arteries prevents or interrupts your heart's blood flow.

Your arteries' walls may eventually develop fatty deposits on them. The fatty deposits are termed atheroma, and the process is known as atherosclerosis.

Lifestyle choices like smoking and binge drinking alcohol on a regular basis can lead to atherosclerosis.

Additionally, having diseases like Diabetes, Hypertension, or High Cholesterol increases your chance of developing atherosclerosis.

Symptoms of Coronary Heart Disease

- Shortness of breath.
- Ache all over the body.
- Dizziness.
- Feeling sick (nausea).
- Angina (chest pain).

However, it is not everyone that exhibits the same symptoms, and some people may not show any symptom before the discovery of coronary heart disease.

Peripheral Arterial Disease

When the arteries leading to the limbs, typically the legs, get blocked, peripheral arterial disease develops. Typically, fatty deposits accumulate in the arteries and impede blood flow to the legs. Other names for it include peripheral vascular disease (PVD).

This may result in: hair loss on the legs and feet, numbness or paralysis in the legs, or cramping leg pain that is worse when walking and improves with rest recurrent leg and foot ulcers (open sores).

Causes of Peripheral Arterial Disease

Peripheral artery disease causes are:

Being a blood vessel disease, PAD is a kind of cardiovascular disease (CVD).

It is typically brought on by an accumulation of fatty deposits in the walls of the arteries in the legs.

Cholesterol and other waste products make up the fatty deposits, or atheroma.

Blood flow to the legs is impeded by the narrowing of the arteries caused by the accumulation of fatty deposits on the artery walls. Atherosclerosis is the name of this process.

Peripheral vascular disease symptoms

Many Peripheral vascular disease sufferers don't exhibit any symptoms. When they walk, some people, however, experience a sharp discomfort in their legs that, in most cases, goes away after a short period of rest. "Intermittent claudication" is the medical word for this condition.

The discomfort, which can be slight to severe, often disappears after a short while when you rest your legs.

Although the discomfort may be greater in one leg, both legs are frequently afflicted at the same time.

Further PAD symptoms

Other PAD examples are:

- Leg numbness or a weakness.

- Hair loss on your legs and feet.

- Weak, slowly expanding toenails.

- Open sores or ulcers on your legs and feet that do not heal.

- Alterations in the color of your legs' skin, such as a bluish or pale tint.

- Smooth skin

- Erectile dysfunction in males.

- Your legs' muscles are thinning (wasting).

The signs of PAD frequently appear gradually over time. If your symptoms appear abruptly or change in intensity, this may indicate a dangerous condition that needs to be treated right once.

Angina (Chest Pain)

Angina, the name for the pain linked to highly severe CHD, typically manifests as a pressure in the chest, arm pain, jaw pain, and other types of discomfort.

A severe angina episode, however, might result in a piercing sensation of tightness or weight, typically in the middle of the chest, which may radiate to the arms, neck, chin, back, or stomach.

Chest discomfort might result from a partial blockage of your coronary arteries (angina). It may be a mildly unpleasant sensation akin to indigestion.

A severe angina episode, however, might result in a piercing sensation of tightness or weight, typically in the middle of the chest, which may radiate to the arms, neck, chin, back, or stomach.

Physical exertion or stressful events might cause angina. The majority of times, symptoms subside in less than 10 minutes, and they may be controlled with rest or a nitrate pill or spray.

Since the form and degree of the angina experience vary greatly from person to person, it is preferable to use the word discomfort rather than pain to describe it. Most people do not regard angina as painful unless it is severe.

In essence, angina is a heart muscle spasm. Physical exertion or stressful events might cause angina.

Chapter Three

The Risk Factors for Heart Diseases

There are a variety of risk factors since cardiovascular disease is such a complicated group of illnesses. The fact that a large number of risk factors for cardiovascular disease interact with each other is an additional problem.

For instance, obesity is a risk factor for type II diabetes as well as being a major risk factor for developing of cardiovascular disease.

As a result, it is difficult to develop any kind of summative formula for predicting cardiovascular illness based on risk factors; the only thing that can be said is that having more risk factors increases your chance of developing a particular type of cardiovascular disease.

The main risk factors for CVD are covered in greater depth below.

Smoking

Smoking raises the risk of coronary heart disease development by two to four times. Smoking increases the risk of sudden cardiac mortality in people with coronary heart disease by around two times compared to non-smokers.

Even non-smokers are at increased risk for heart disease due to exposure to secondhand smoke, according to the British Heart Foundation, who estimates that such exposure can raise the risk of coronary heart disease by up to 25%. Cigarette smoking has a significant impact on other risk variables.

Smoking raises the risk of heart disease through pretty well-understood pathways. The primary danger is related to smokers' greater propensity for thrombosis, which can result in myocardial infarction.

Increased atherosclerosis, blood pressure, heart rate, cardiac output, and coronary blood flow are other processes.

Smoking also raises carbon monoxide levels in the body, which bind to hemoglobin and reduce oxygen delivery to bodily tissues. Around 1 billion men and 250 million women are estimated to smoke every day globally.

Obesity

Even in the absence of any additional risk factors, obesity, especially in individuals with extra fat around the waist, raises the risk of Cardiovascular Disease.

Weight gain makes the heart work harder, increases blood pressure, cholesterol, and triglyceride levels, and decreases HDL (High Density Lipoprotein) cholesterol levels.

Atherosclerosis and thrombolytic embolism risk can both be elevated by all of these causes. Type II diabetes, another risk factor for cardiovascular disease, is also more likely to develop as a result.

Diabetes

An individual's capacity to maintain a healthy blood glucose level is impacted by diabetes. Type I and Type II diabetes are the two variations of the illness. Insulin-dependent diabetes, another name for type I diabetes, is brought on by a lack of insulin production in the body.

The more prevalent kind of diabetes, type II, is brought on by either insufficient insulin production by the body or improper insulin processing by the cells.

Through elevated cholesterol levels, hypertension, and atherosclerosis, each of these kinds can raise the chance of developing cardiovascular disease. Heart disease and insulin resistance are connected.

According to World Health Organisation (WHO) projections, there are more than 180 million diabetics in the globe, and by 2030, that number is expected to more than double.

High Blood Pressure

Cardiovascular and vascular system illnesses are both closely associated with high blood pressure (hypertension).

Due to the heart having to work harder to pump blood, high blood pressure affects it, causing it to thicken and stiffen; this can result in heart attacks.

Pressure on the walls of the vasculature has an impact on the circulatory system and can cause aneurisms and stroke.

One in four persons in the United States has been diagnosed with hypertension, a decrease from the 1980s when the incidence was almost one in two. High blood pressure is a major issue in industrialized nations.

High levels of Low Density Lipoprotein (LDL) Cholesterol

Low density lipoprotein cholesterol (LDL) primarily raises the risk of cardiovascular disease by causing an increase in atherosclerotic fatty plaque buildup in blood vessels. As opposed to what was previously believed, recent findings indicate that this is a more active process, with LDL cholesterol actually activating endothelial cells to express adhesion molecules that hasten atherosclerosis.

In general, cholesterol levels have been growing worldwide, and estimates indicate that this trend will continue up to 2030 (interestingly, levels are predicted to decline in North America and Western Europe).

Additional risk factors for Cardiovascular Diseases

Other risk factors have a significant role in the development of CVD. Sedentary lifestyle, for instance, is considered to be a major risk factor.

In addition to lowering cholesterol and obesity, physical activity makes the heart and muscles work harder to circulate blood throughout the body.

Another risk factor is alcohol use, which is complicated since moderate consumption can lower the risk of heart disease (due to antioxidant polyphenols that prevent LDL cholesterol from oxidizing), while heavy consumption actually raises the risk of CHD and stroke (by increasing blood pressure).

Nutrition is another important risk factor that is frequently mentioned. A poor diet directly affects the body's fat concentrations, which raises the risk of high cholesterol and obesity, the blood sugar level, which raises the risk of type II diabetes, and the blood salt level, which raises the risk of blood pressure and stroke.

Heart Problems in Men

On average, males have heart disease a decade earlier than women. Erectile dysfunction is another early warning symptom that few people may overlook. "Heart issues frequently predict sexual difficulties."

Positively, any risk factor that draws your attention, including Erectile Dysfunction, can lead to better preventative care.

Many people mistakenly believe that erectile dysfunction is defined as the inability to achieve or maintain an erection for long enough to engage in satisfying sexual activity.

In reality, however, erectile dysfunction is more often than not the result of a physical issue rather than an age-related condition.

The fact that the penis, like the heart, is a vascular organ is one of the main reasons erectile dysfunction is seen as an indicator for general cardiovascular health.

Since the arteries in the penis is considerably smaller than those in the heart, arterial damage manifests there first, sometimes years before heart disease symptoms.

An 80% chance of getting heart problems within 10 years exists for men in their 40s who have erection issues but no other cardiovascular disease risk factors.

Also, low testosterone levels are sometimes mistaken for just having less sex desire, but they are also known to be associated with heart disease and type 2 diabetes. According to research, low testosterone might be regarded as a metabolic and cardiovascular risk factor.

Low testosterone is frequently present in individuals with metabolic syndrome or abdominal obesity.

Diabetes and metabolic syndrome are the two main risk factors for heart disease, along with excessive blood sugar, abnormal cholesterol levels, and excess belly fat. The total picture of cardiac risk does not only include low testosterone.

Again, stress, fury, and anxiety can reduce blood flow to the heart by increasing blood pressure and stress hormone levels. Some harm may manifest right away. For instance, your risk of a heart attack is roughly five times higher and your risk of stroke is three times higher in the two hours following an angry outburst.

Over time, the consequences of ongoing stress can compound and harm arteries. Heart disease is more likely to affect men, particularly those who are unpleasant or irritable. Heart disease-related sexual issues may exacerbate worry or strain on relationships. Stress can also have an impact on sleep, which has an impact on heart health.

When it comes to heart health, physical, emotional, and psychological variables are all connected. Men who experience persistent stress, sadness, or anxiety have to get a baseline assessment of all the risk factors for developing heart disease.

Heart Disease in Women

In the US, the top cause of mortality for women is cardiovascular disease. Heart disease kills seven times more women than breast cancer, a fact that many women are unaware of.

In 2018, 300,977 women died from heart disease. Comparatively, 283,721 people died from cancer overall, 42,455 of them from breast cancer.

Every illness merits consideration, awareness, and action. However, you won't know you need to learn more about heart disease if you don't aware it poses such a significant danger. And you might put off starting to take precautions to lower your risk.

According to one study, just 50% of women under the age of 55 who experienced a heart attack believed they were at risk before the event. Yet several risk factors existed for those same ladies. They were simply ignorant.

The severe chest discomfort that is a traditional sign of a heart attack in males doesn't affect many women. Some report feeling breathless or drained of all energy. Other unusual symptoms include nausea as well as discomfort in the shoulders, neck, and abdomen.

In one research, women described having severe weariness and having trouble sleeping up to two months in advance of having a heart attack.

Only roughly one in eight women had chest discomfort during a heart attack, and even then, they did not characterize it as pain but rather as pressure, hurting, or tightness.

Certain examples proof that women can suffer heart problems:

Diabetes

Women are more likely to develop heart disease than males are, maybe because women with diabetes are more likely to be affected by additional risk factors such obesity, hypertension, and high cholesterol.

Diabetes negates the fact that women typically get heart disease 10 years later than men do. Diabetes doubles the risk of a second heart attack and raises the chance of heart failure in women who have already experienced a heart attack.

Cigarette Smoking

Smoking increases the risk of heart attack in women more than it does in men. Additionally, women are less likely to succeed in stopping, and those who do are more likely to relapse.

Additionally, women might not find nicotine replacement as helpful, and since the menstrual period impacts the symptoms of cigarette withdrawal, they can have uneven outcomes with anti-smoking drugs.

Metabolic Disorder

This set of health issues, which includes having a big waist circumference, high blood pressure, glucose intolerance, low HDL cholesterol, and high triglycerides, raises your risk of getting diabetes, heart disease, and stroke.

According to research, metabolic syndrome is the main risk factor for women who get heart attacks at an extremely young age.

In patients receiving bypass surgery, metabolic syndrome increased the chance of death within eight years for women more than it did for males.

Lipid in the Blood

A woman's natural estrogen helps shield her against heart disease prior to menopause by raising High density Lipoprotein (good) cholesterol and lowering Low Density Lipoprotein LDL (bad) cholesterol.

Women had greater overall cholesterol levels than males do after menopause. However, this may not fully account for the abrupt increase in heart disease risk following menopause.

Increased triglycerides are a significant factor in women's cardiovascular risk. The risk of dying from heart disease in women over 65 seems to be only increased by low High density Lipoprotein HDL and high triglycerides.

In what ways does the Cardiovascular System in Men and Women Differ?

Numerous sex-related variations in the cardiovascular system have been discovered by researchers. These subtle variations, which frequently occur on a microscopic level, can have an impact on how men and women develop heart disease. Several instances include:

Blood count: Red blood cells are smaller in females. Women are thus less able to take in or carry about as much oxygen at once.

Hormones: In contrast to testosterone in men, estrogen and progesterone predominate in women. Numerous elements of heart well-being and overall health can be impacted by these hormones.

Anatomy: Women's hearts and blood vessels are smaller. Additionally, their ventricles' walls are thinner.

Changes to cardiovascular systems: Women are more affected than males by changes in altitude or body posture (such as rising up rapidly after lying down). Intense dips in blood pressure or fainting are more common in women.

Chapter Four

How do alkaline diets work?

All biological fluids and tissues have a pH that is closely controlled within a very narrow range.

Each type of cell, tissue, and organ, including the blood, muscles, and stomach, has a certain optimum pH level. Acid-alkaline balance or acid-alkaline homeostasis is the process of keeping pH levels within a certain range.

Alkaline foods have a tonic effect on the body. Blood acidity is balanced by alkaline meals, which gives the body a breath of fresh air and helps the body regenerate and repair damaged cells.

Faster cell oxidation caused by acid-rich foods produces acid bombs that circulate in the bloodstream and cause havoc with the body.

Alkaline diets are ones that fully forbid any foods that include acids. They are sometimes referred to as "electric meals" since they assist the body's natural capacity for self-repair. They just exist naturally; they are not modified, hybridized, or exposed to radiation.

Increased absorption of iron, copper, and other essential vitamins and minerals that support the immune system are made possible by alkaline foods.

They are foods that increase your blood's alkalinity, which wards against diseases and infections because many bacteria prefer an acidic environment to live in.

Maintaining appropriate blood pH levels can be made easier by identifying meals that have an alkalizing effect on the body.

The phrase "alkaline diet" describes an eating regimen that emphasizes providing the body with the nutrients and sustenance it needs to be healthy, active, and vibrant.

People who have stronger immunity, more energy, and reduced discomfort are benefits of an enhanced acid-alkaline balance in their body.

Alkaline diets enhanced bone health by lowering osteoporosis and arthritic pain, digestion, and gastrointestinal discomfort from ulcers, bowel problems, and acid reflux, increased nutrient absorption, and enhanced detoxification by balancing the body's pH equilibrium.

Humans can recover from any chronic illness when their blood has a "normal or slightly alkaline pH."

What Benefits Can an Alkaline Diet Offer?

The benefits of an alkaline diet include:

1. It is extremely low in fat, which guards against heart disease and other cardiac issues.
2. Free of cholesterol.
3. It is devoid of alcohol.
4. It prevents and treats cancer.
5. Both prevents and treats stroke.
6. Herpes simplex virus treatment and prevention
7. Reduces and prevents high blood pressure.
8. It has very low saturated fat content, reducing the risk of developing significant cardiac conditions.
9. It has no refined sugar.
10. Diabetes is treated and prevented.

11. Ensure that the majority of program participants lose weight.

What Foods Should You Avoid on an Alkaline Diet?

A complete alkaline diet plan forgoes many items that are not naturally acidic. The bulk of the food you consume has a high acidity, which hinders the body's capacity to heal and recover. On an alkaline diet, you can't eat:

- Alcoholic drinks.
- Soy and products made from soy.
- Corn.
- Dairy items.
- Sugar.
- Meat from poultry.
- Vitamin and mineral supplements in food
- Garlic.
- Fruits grown with genetically altered organisms.
- Fish and seafood.
- Colors and flavors.
- A variety of meats.

- Eggs.

- Prepared foods

- Cans of fruit.

- Fruits that are seedless.

- Foods containing baking powder or other substances, such as yeast.

- Wheat.

- Fast meals.

- Plants that have been genetically engineered.

How to Get Rid of Disease-Causing Substances and Prevent Symptoms

We must first learn how to "remove the cause" because the majority of debilitating ailments developed as a result of self-generated toxins caused by undigested meals.

This only suggests that we should stop eating "acid-forming meals," which turn our bodily tissue acidic and impair our cells' capacity to absorb oxygen.

The primary underlying cause of the majority of ailments is acid-producing diets. We must first comprehend the principles of how to accomplish it in order to treat the root of the problem and its symptoms.

Low quality, toxic body cells weaken your immune system's ability to protect and defend itself against all causes and situations of disease; understanding how to treat these reasons will help you avoid this.

Learn how to eat alkaline foods, quit eating meals that cause acidity, and live a toxin-free life.

Some Alkaline Fruits and Veggies that can Help You

Alkaline Vegetables

Arame, Wild, Arugula, Cherry and Plum Tomato, Cucumber, Wakame, Lettuce except for the Iceberg, Nori, Watercress, Tomatillo, Turnip Greens, Onions, Squash, Okra, Hijiki, Purslane, Verdolaga, Avocado, Izote flower and leaf, Kale, Mushrooms except for Shitake, Bell Pepper, Chayote, Zucchini, Nopales, Olives, Dulse, Garbanzo Beans, Dandelion Greens, and Amaranth.

Alkaline Fruits

Soft Jelly Coconuts, Papayas, Melons, Figs, Grapes, Sour sups, Prunes, Bananas, Apples, Pears, Limes, Prickly Pear, Cherries, Orange, Currants, Rasins, Peaches, Plums, Mango, Berries, Dates, and Cantaloupe.

Alkaline Grains

Fonio, Rye Tef, Kamut, Amaranth, Quinoa, Wild Rice, and Spelt.

Alkaline Spices and Seasonings

Dill, Achiote, Habanero, Sage, Savory, Basil, Thyme, Bay Leaf Cayenne Cloves, Onion Powder, Sweet Basil, Pure Sea Salt, Oregano, Powdered Granulated Seaweed and Tarragon.

Alkaline Herbs

Chamomile, Fennel, Red Raspberry, Elderberry & Tila Dill, Onion powder, Basil, Cayenne, Ginger, Burdock, Oregano…and many more.

Chapter Five

Heart Diseases and Treatment Approach

There are different traditional methods used in the treatment of heart problems, as there are different types of heart problems with different causes.

In the course of writing this book, I will show you different methods such as the use of therapeutic alkaline herbs, the employment of physiotherapy especially for stroke patients and the consumption of healing diets that contains reduced amount of fat, cholesterol and acid contents.

The first step to this treatment is detoxification. Detoxification helps the body to get rid of substances (such as fatty deposits, toxins, excess acid…and more) that are accumulated in the body.

The herbs that can be used for detoxification are:

Stinging nettle root, Nopal plant, Sea moss plant, Elderberry, Linden leaf and Burdock root.

Take care to thoroughly clean this plant under running water after gathering them. To dry them, place them directly in the sun.

Preparing the Herbs

- Ensure that the plants are entirely dry before storing them in a dry, sterile container.
- Pulverize them to a fine powder.
- Mix one tablespoon of each of the aforementioned herbs with two glasses of alkaline or spring water.
- Place it close to a source of heat and wait for it to boil.
- After three minutes of boiling, or when you see the phytoconstituents are starting to emerge and the water's color has changed, remove from heat.
- Simply remove the herb from the heater and let it cool down for a couple of minutes before consumption, even though it is ideal to consume herbs hot so the bitterness will be reduced.

- One cup of the herb should be taken in the morning and night for two weeks.

Throughout this process, you can also consume a broad range of other fruits and vegetables, including watermelon, berries, mushrooms, zucchini, cactus plants, and leafy greens. Additional choices include tamarind juice and water. You are not required to eat any solid meals during these two weeks of detoxification, even if they are on the dietary lists. Grains, nuts, and seeds are not permitted foods. When the treatment process is over, you can consume them.

Benefits Alkaline Detoxifying Herbs Provide

The aforementioned herbs help the body with the following tasks:

- Body rejuvenation.
- Remove poisons from bodily waste.
- Removes excess body fat.

- Cells in the body proliferate.

- Stimulates and purifies the blood.

Heart Problems Treated with Alkaline Therapeutic Herbs

Since the dawn of civilization, herbs have been utilized as medicines. Patients with congestive heart failure, systolic hypertension, angina pectoris, atherosclerosis, cerebral insufficiency, venous insufficiency, arrhythmia…and more have all benefited from herbal therapy for cardiovascular illnesses.

However, many of the herbal medicines now in use have not received thorough scientific evaluation, and some might have substantial adverse consequences and significant medication interactions.

Herbs have always played a significant role in society and have been highly regarded for their therapeutic benefits. Digitoxin from Digitalis purpurea (foxglove), salicin (the aspirin source) from Salix alba (willow bark), and reserpine from Rauwolfia serpentina (snakeroot), Ephedrine from Ephedra sinica (ma-huang), to name a few, are just a few examples of the numerous contributions made by herbal medicine to the commercial drug preparations produced today.

Herbs for Angina Treatment

Hawthorn (Crataegus species)

A variety of Crataegus species, including Crataegus oxyacantha, Crataegus monogyna, and Crataegus pinnatifida in the West and Crataegus pinnatifida in China, are collectively referred to as Crataegus hawthorn.

This name has gained recognition in contemporary herbal literature as a vital tonic for the cardiovascular system that is especially helpful for angina.

Oligomeric procyanins, flavonoids, and catechins are only a few of the physiologically active compounds found in Crataegus leaves, flowers, and fruits. According to recent research, Crataegus extract can suppress the production of thromboxane and has antioxidant qualities.

Additionally, when rats are fed a hyperlipidemic diet, Crataegus extract counteracts the rise in cholesterol, triglyceride, and phospholipid levels in low-density lipoprotein (LDL) and very low-density lipoprotein; this suggests that it may slow the development of atherosclerosis.

Additionally, Crataegus reduces cholesterol buildup in the liver by accelerating cholesterol conversion to bile acids and inhibiting cholesterol production.

Another study found that large doses of Crataegus extract have cardioprotective effects on ischemic-reperfused hearts without increasing coronary blood flow.

In short, Crataegus has a modest hypotensive impact, enhances coronary perfusion, inhibits atherogenesis, and has both positive inotropic and negative chronotropic effects.

A Crataegus extract was shown in a research to significantly enhance cardiac function in individuals with New York Heart Association class II heart failure. Systolic blood pressure divided by heart rate was the study's key parameters of analysis.

Hawthorn hardly has any negative consequences. In fact, Crataegus has a possibly lower arrhythmogenic risk than other inotropic medications like epinephrine, amrinone, milrinone, and digoxin because it can lengthen the effective refractory period, whereas the other treatments all shorten this parameter.

Salvia miltiorrhiza

Salvia miltiorrhiza (dan-shen), a Chinese native and a close cousin of the Western sage Salvia officinalis The root of S miltiorrhiza is a sedative, cooling, and circulatory stimulant used in traditional Chinese medicine.

Salvia miltiorrhiza has been demonstrated to widen coronary arteries in all doses, much as P notoginseng, suggesting that it may be beneficial as an antianginal medication.

Additionally, depending on its concentration, S miltiorrhiza has a varying effect on other arteries, which makes it less likely to be effective in treating hypertension.

On ischemic myocardium, Salvia miltiorrhiza appears to have a protective effect, accelerating the restoration of contractile force after reoxygenation.

Due to its free radical-scavenging properties, S miltiorrhiza has recently been demonstrated to protect cardiac mitochondrial membranes against ischemia-reperfusion damage and lipid peroxidation.

Herbs for Atherosclerosis Treatment
Garlic (*Allium sativum*)

Garlic (*Allium sativum*) has long been prized for its therapeutic qualities in addition to its usage in meals. One natural remedy that has been studied more thoroughly by the scientific community is garlic.

The use of garlic to reduce atherosclerosis has garnered a lot of attention in recent decades. Garlic has been shown to have several positive cardiovascular benefits, much like many of the other herbal remedies previously mentioned.

These benefits, which include decreasing blood pressure, preventing platelet aggregation, improving fibrinolytic activity, lowering serum cholesterol and triglyceride levels, and preserving the elastic characteristics of the aorta, have been shown in several investigations.

It has been demonstrated that consuming substantial amounts of fresh garlic (0.25 to 1.0 g/kg, or around 5-20 average-sized 4-g cloves in a person weighing 78.7 kg) results in the positive benefits indicated above.

Additionally, the blood pressure-lowering effects of garlic in hypertensive individuals have been investigated.

Moderate garlic use has little negative effects other than a smell on the breath and body. However, eating more than five cloves per day may cause heartburn, flatulence, and other gastrointestinal problems. Garlic has been linked to allergic responses in certain persons, most often allergic contact dermatitis.

Peripheral and Cerebral Vascular Disease

Ginkgo biloba **(maidenhair tree)**

Ginkgo biloba (maidenhair tree), which has been around for more than 200 million years, appears to have been spared from extinction by humans since it is still alive in Far Eastern temple gardens while being extinct in the West for millennia. In 1730, it was brought back to Europe and quickly became a popular decorative tree.

G. biloba extract contains at least two categories of constituents that have positive pharmacological effects. The flavonoids act as free radical scavengers and decrease capillary permeability and fragility. Without significantly influencing blood pressure, the terpenes (i.e., ginkgolides) block platelet-activating factor, lower vascular resistance, and enhance circulatory flow.

It is used to treat cerebral inadequacy and its impact on vertigo, tinnitus, memory, and mood, according to study. Additionally, it seems to be effective in treating peripheral vascular disorders, such as intermittent claudication and diabetic retinopathy.

According to study, it can considerably reduce the ischemia in the muscles during exercise as indicated by the transcutaneous partial pressure of oxygen. It may be beneficial in the treatment of intermittent claudication and peripheral artery disease in broad sense due to its quick anti-ischemic activity.

Herbs for Hypertension Treatment
Rauwolfia serpentina (snakeroot)

Hindu Ayurvedic medicine has long used the root of R serpentina (snakeroot), the natural source of the alkaloid reserpine.

R. serpentina root was originally used to treat hypertension and psychoses in 1931, according to Indian literature.

One of the first medications to be used extensively to treat systemic hypertension was reserpine. It works by permanently preventing biogenic amines (such as norepinephrine, dopamine, and serotonin) from entering the storage vesicles of central and peripheral adrenergic neurons, leaving the catecholamines vulnerable to degradation by intraneuronal monoamine oxidase in the cytoplasm.

By reducing cardiac output, peripheral vascular resistance, heart rate, and renin production, reserpine reduces blood pressure. The usage of reserpine has decreased as a result of the development of alternative antihypertensive medications with less side effects on the central nervous system.

Reserpine should be taken orally once in a day at doses of 0.25 mg or less, or even 0.05 mg when combined with a diuretic. The typical adult dosage using the entire root is 50 to 200 mg/d given once daily or in two separate doses.

The use of *Rauwolfia* alkaloids is not advised in those who have previously shown sensitivity to them, have a history of mental illness, particularly if they have suicidal thoughts, have active ulcerative colitis or peptic ulcer disease, or are undergoing electroconvulsive treatment.

Sedation and the inability to focus and handle difficult activities are the most frequent side effects. Reserpine usage must be stopped at the first symptom of depression since it can create mental depression, which can occasionally lead to suicide.

Other herbs for hypertension are:

i.   Hand flower plant (Flor de Manita).

ii.   Dandelion greens.

iii.   Burdock root.

iv.   Rye plant.

Hand flower plant (Flor de Manita)

Mexican plant known as the "hand flower plant," or "Flor de Manita," is mostly used to treat heart-related conditions. Both low and high blood pressure can be effectively treated with this herb. This indicates that it has a highly effective component that can maintain blood pressure levels.

With the usage of this herb, the blood cholesterol level is maintained, and it also helps with the treatment of cardiovascular health issues.

Green Dandelion

Dandelion is naturally diuretic, which means it enhances both the frequency and quality of urination. As a result, it helps to reduce blood pressure. This is due to the fact that urinating is one of the best ways to lower blood pressure.

Burdock Root

Although it is not well recognized, burdock tea can lower blood pressure levels. High potassium levels in burdock help to relax the veins and arteries and ease stress in the heart and circulatory system.

As a result, it aids in reducing the risk of heart attacks, strokes, atherosclerosis (a condition in which plaque builds up inside the arteries), and many other cardiovascular issues.

Rye plant

The rye plant is a well-known heart-healthy herb that may be consumed regularly. Magnesium, which promotes heart health and controls blood pressure, is abundant in it. Additionally, it has a lot of soluble fiber, which helps lower cholesterol.

Preparation of Herbs and Dosages

- Rinse each plant individually to remove any dirt.
- After the herbs are dried, powder them.

- Place them in various lidded containers to keep moisture off of them.
- Mix 3–4 cups of alkaline or spring water with half a teaspoon of each of the herbs.
- Place in your pot and bring to a boil for four to five minutes.
- Make sure the contents are emptied into the water before removing it from the heat; this will cause a change in the water's color.
- Turn off the heat and let it cool.
- Drain food before eating.
- Until you are fully well, these herbs should be taken in the morning and at night.

Physiotherapy Solution for Heart Problems

Physiotherapy is a branch of alternative medicine that uses physical manipulation to improve a patient's mobility, function, and overall well-being.

Physical rehabilitation, injury prevention, health and fitness are all benefits of physiotherapy. Physiotherapists engage you in your own healing.

When combined with regular medical care, chest physiotherapy is more successful than medical care alone at reducing discomfort and dyspnea and removing chest secretions.

When combined with medical treatment, the estimated benefit of cardiac rehabilitation programs in CAD patients is around nearly twice more than when medical treatment is used solely.

Physiotherapists commonly employed the manual approach and postural drainage; however, patients with serious cardiovascular disease are thought to have a relative adverse reaction to head-down postural drainage. In a healthy adult, a brief session of 30 degree head-down postural drainage can reduce heart rate, mean arterial blood pressure, and diastolic duration.

The following can be done by a Physiotherapist:

- Intermittent positive pressure respiration breathing exercises: Any negative effects at this point are carefully observed since breathing exercises promote venous return and intermittent positive pressure respiration lowers venous return.

- The massaging of the calves to lower the risk of deep vein thrombosis.
- Self-induced relaxation to lessen emotional tension.
- Reckless footwork. (Vigorous foot motion` is highly recommended). The first therapy should be sitting with assistance.

The exercises listed below are done while sitting with assistance.

- Each foot actively adducts and abducts.
- Active foot flexion and extension.
- Each leg's flexion and extension.

The next exercises are done while lying down. In cardiac work, lying down is an improvement to sitting since doing so increases venous return.

- Lie on your side. Leg entrapment
- Frequently lying. Leg elongation

- Lying when supine. Each knee contracts its quadriceps.

In addition to the aforementioned exercises, which are performed daily for a week, the patient may sit up in bed for about half-hour and use a wheelchair to use the restroom.

Two people should lift patients into and out of beds. The cardiac output is believed to rise by about 40% when getting out of bed requires effort.

- Up to two hours may be spent sitting up in bed.
- The patient is permitted to move round the bed.
- The patient is free to move about the space in the room
- The patient can go to the restroom on foot.

Waistline Exercise

1. Stand straight and slant backwards with your feet apart and your arms extended over your head. Six times, up to twenty times.
2. Make full circles with your upper body starting from your hips while standing straight with your

71

feet apart and your hands behind your neck. Two circles in one direction, followed by two in the opposite. 10 circles are added on each side as you go.

Breathing Exercise

- While sitting, raise different leg six times. Gradually progress to 20 times.
- While Side lying, abduct each leg 10 times. Gradually progress to 20 times.

Alkaline Diet for Healthy Heart

There are many available alkaline diets that can help you manage your heart very well. These diets can be prepared with the employment of the items in the alkaline food list.

You can get some of the alkaline diets in my book called Dr. Sebi Lung Diseases Alkaline Diet And Herbs (Esther Gbemy) and Natural Alkaline Diets, Water & Medicinal Herbs for Herpes (Esther Gbemy).

References

Edward Nason. An overview of cardiovascular disease and research. WR-467-RS January 2007.

Ezzati, Lopez, Rodgers and Murray (2004) Comparative Quantification of Health Risks: Global and Regional Burden of Disease Attribution to Selected Major Risk Factors, World Health Organisation, Chapter 7.Availableat:http://www.who.int/publications/cra/chapters/volume1 /0391-0496.

Ganjia, Kamannaa and Kashyap (2003) Niacin and cholesterol: role in cardiovascular disease (review), The Journal of Nutritional Biochemistry, 114:6 , 298-305

Rosemary Samios. Physiotherapy In A Coronary Care Unit. School of Physiotherapy Aust. J.. Physiother., XVII, 2, Jnne, 1971.

Smith, Fischer and Sears (2000) "Environmental Tobacco Smoke, Cardiovascular Disease, and the Nonlinear Dose-Response Hypothesis", Toxicological Sciences, 554, 462-472.